I0449241

Common Sense Keto: How I Lost 88 Pounds

Christina D. Ford

Published by Christina Ford, 2019.

FIRST EDITION

www.christinadford.com

Table of Contents

Dedication.. 1

Introduction.. 3

Disclaimer... 11

What is the Keto Diet, Anyway?.................................. 13

What Do You Mean, No Bread?!............................... 17

Electrolyte City 21

Food Lists 23

Simple Rules for Grocery Shopping 31

Mealtime Hacks 35

Eating Out... 39

Keto Happy Hour... 41

Cheater, Cheater 45

Fasts.. 49

Intermittent Fasting 53

Recap 55

Seven-Day Meal Plan 59

Dedication

When considering who I would dedicate this book to, I had several thoughts. I thought about the people who encouraged me, the people who complimented me, and the people who have endlessly asked that I put my journey into words on paper so they could read it and show their friends.

I came to a final conclusion pretty quickly.

I dedicate this book to myself, in the name of self-love.

Self-love is something I've struggled with my whole life. I can also honestly say that I have no one to thank more than myself. I did the work. I put in the time. I prepped, prepared, and stayed on track and have kept the weight off of my body for over two years.

I am sincerely grateful for every step I have taken that has lead me here, to the point of sharing my journey with others, and it is so empowering to claim my own appreciation for my efforts.

Introduction

As I sit here contemplating how to open this book in an engaging, humorous, authentic way, I imagine myself in a room full of regular men and women, brought together by a problem that plagues millions – our struggle to lose weight.

I'm sitting in the back of the room in one of those hard backed plastic chairs that has that wicked curve that a spine should never be put against. Uncomfortable, I shyly stand up, wave to all of you after almost tripping over my big feet on my way to the podium, and say "Hi, I'm Christina, and I'm a recovering carboholic."

This is the part where you all respond in monotone "Hi, Christina."

Now we have met. I can begin by telling my story, exposing my very overweight past.

A part of me has felt at war with my body for a very, very long time. I was brought up by a generation of "clean your plate" parents in the South, where almost all foods are fried, including the vegetables. Portion size and nutrition were never discussed half as much as how you could save bacon grease to fry chicken the next day, and meat and potatoes were included with every meal. Some form of bread was always available, from biscuits to cornbread.

Don't get me wrong; I'm not knocking it. These are some of my favorite foods, the most flavorful and yummy meals in existence.

They also immediately bring to mind family and a sense of home. It was soul food, the kind that sat heavy in your belly and made you feel warm and happy and loved.

There was only one problem that developed rather fast.

I was hungry all the time, so I ate A LOT.

I was bigger than most of the girls in my high school graduating class, not incredibly overweight but not slender either. I was soft around the edges, but I didn't mind it much. I was just bigger-boned and broader shouldered than most of the other girls. Or at least, that was what I told myself.

After high school, I went on to college. Food became a matter of convenience, something to jam in around class, studying, and working a part-time job. The dining hall had waffles every day for breakfast, noodles for lunch, mac and cheese for dinner. My dorm room had a stockpile of ramen, soda, and microwave meals. I put on the freshman fifteen just like everyone else. Then it climbed to twenty, followed by thirty.

Weight climbing higher than it ever had, I started counting calories and exercising, taking Karate classes six times a week. It stopped the gain, but I didn't lose anything. I had muscle tone, but I was still overweight according to my doctor and the dreaded body mass index (BMI) chart. The karate helped with my confidence, but never moved the scale. I couldn't understand it, but I was assured that I was healthy, just a bit overweight.

Two years later, I met my soon to be husband, and one month before we tied the knot, we discovered that yes, birth control pills do fail, and I became pregnant. This led to a lot of joy, and an additional 55 pounds onto my body as late night cravings for spaghetti became a nightly occurrence.

I tried everything, and I do mean *everything*, to lose weight after my daughter was born. There was not a pill on any store shelf I hadn't tried, an exercise regime I hadn't subjected myself to, a weight loss plan that required weekly meetings and weigh-ins that I hadn't attended. For all of my efforts, I lost no more than ten pounds.

Five years later, I got pregnant again. Another 15 pounds was layered on, and I kid you not, at this point I had made friends with my fat. It seemed like nothing I did worked anyway, so I just gave up trying. Or at least, I gave up until the only stores I could shop at had multiple x's in front of the sizes. Depressed, I'd try again. Inevitably, I'd fail again.

Why am I telling you all of this? Because I want you to know you aren't alone. I know I'm not the only one who feels like they have tried it all with little success. I know, without a doubt, if you are reading this book that you have tried and tried and tried until you are flat tired of trying.

I know you're sick to death of being uncomfortable in your own skin, because I sure was.

Here's something else you should know about me, though. I am really, really stubborn. There's something to that – it fuels my willpower.

Close to the end of 2017, topping out at my highest weight ever at 275 pounds, I went in for my yearly visit to the doctor and was told that I was not only obese, but morbidly obese, and showing signs of pre-diabetes.

I was terrified. Diabetes can wreak havoc on your entire body. I decided, right then and there, that I was not going to let that happen.

I was honest with my doctor about my attempts to lose weight. At the time, I was barely eating 1,200 calories per day, a large caloric deficit that should have had me shedding pounds! Yet, the scale never moved. My doctor agreed that I technically should be losing weight, but didn't offer any real solutions for why I wasn't.

Frustrated, but not ready to give in to a possibly life-altering diagnosis, I set about learning about nutrition for the first time in my life. I read everything I could find before finally stumbling across an article that mentioned that pre-diabetes is a sign of insulin resistance. As in, my pancreas was giving up on regulating my blood sugar. It was simply worn out by the way I fed my body. I went on to discover that blood sugar is highly affected by carbohydrates.

Easy peasy, right? I looked up diets that cut out carbohydrates and found the Keto Diet almost immediately. I also found another surprising tidbit of information. Weight loss is mostly about what you eat, and less about exercise. Of course, exercise is important, but at this point the tiniest bit of exercise had my knees swollen and aching for days. I decided to diet first and get some of the excess weight off my joints before I considered a regular exercise regimen.

After a quick call to my doctor to ensure the diet was a safe option for me, I received the go-ahead to begin the diet as long as I scheduled a follow-up appointment in 30 days.

I picked a date to start, got prepared to cut restrict my carb intake for fourteen days, and crossed my fingers. Two weeks later, I had lost 15 pounds.

I couldn't believe it. I'd never had results come so quickly. Excited that something was FINALLY working, I decided to continue on and learn as I went. By the time I had my 30-day checkup, I was down 22 pounds total. My doctor was really encouraging, and after some questions about how I was feeling and some other tests, he gave me the go-ahead to continue.

That was beginning of my journey. To date, I have lost 88 pounds using the Keto diet. The weight flew off me at first, and has slowed as I have approached my goal weight, which is a nice, healthy 165 pounds.

Now, considering that I'm 5'6", 165 pounds still makes for a slightly overweight BMI, yes, I am aware.

Guess how much I care?

Nada. That BMI chart can suck my big toe. I chose that as my goal weight because it strikes a balance for me between super skinny, which I don't aspire to be, and slightly curvy, which I like quite a bit. I wanted to find something that felt right for ME.

I'm not quite there yet. I, like you, am still a work in progress. I am only just beginning to explore exercise now that my knees are bearing less weight. This also means that my weight loss slows, because I am working on building muscle.

I'm okay with that. It's really not about the number on the scale, y'all. It's all about how I feel about myself.

I currently weigh in at 187 pounds, and wear a size 11/12, compared to the size 22's when I was nearing close to 300 pounds.

I managed to accomplish this through constant trial and error. There was so much information out there, and I spent hours and hours of my life digging through countless sources of information, from consulting my physician, to reading books, scouring magazine articles, cruising the internet, joining social media groups – there wasn't a single stone I left unturned in my attempt to save myself from diabetes and a host of other medical issues that would have surely followed.

I also quickly found that most people, no matter how inspired by my success, just didn't want to do that kind of research for themselves. I mean, honestly, to anyone just starting out, that seems like a lot of work!

Let's be real. Most of us are super busy people, and we have other things to think about besides our diet!

That's where my idea for this little guidebook comes in. This is my no-nonsense, practical guide that I used to lose weight with Keto. I'm laying out all my tips and tricks, including my cheat days where I ate whatever the heck I wanted, and how I managed that without derailing my progress. I'm going to lay out everything I know, because everywhere I go, every time I run into an old acquaintance, I get asked repeatedly – How did you do it?!

This little book is the answer to that question.

It's really, really nice to meet you all.

Toodaloo,

Christina D. Ford, Former Carboholic

Disclaimer

I have written this book of my personal journey with weight loss to the best of my ability; however, it is important to note that I am not a physician. I am not able to give you medical advice. The general information included in this book is not intended to be used as a substitute for medical advice. I strongly encourage you to discuss any dietary and supplement changes that you wish to make with a qualified medical professional beforehand to make sure that it will not cause any new or exacerbate any existing medical issues you may have.

The primary purpose of this book is to share information based upon my own personal experiences and preferences. The use of this information is at the sole choice and risk of the reader.

Please take good care of yourself.

What is the Keto Diet, Anyway?

In a nutshell, the Keto Diet is a low carbohydrate, moderate protein, and high fat diet. Eating this way alters the metabolic state of the body, and is commonly referred to as ketosis. Ketosis is a switch for the body from its reliance on carbohydrates for energy to using ketones for energy instead, which is what is produced when the liver processes the new high fat portion of the diet.

How's that for an info-dump?

Now, listen Bob, don't get hung up on the word "Diet". A diet is just a specific way of eating. I could honestly call my former carb-loving life a diet. It was how I ate, it was what I ate, and it was what it did to my body.

I had to do some serious thinking around the word "diet" myself.

Have you ever noticed people trying to rename the word "Diet"? That's where the word "lifestyle" enters the picture. I'd pick up a magazine where someone would go about describing their brand new "lifestyle".

That's fantastic for you, I'd think, skimming it over.

Yet, I had resistance over that word, too A "lifestyle" change seemed to imply that I needed to change my life. While I certainly believed that losing weight would change certain aspects of my life, I already really loved my life as it was. I was really, truly grateful for a lot of things. I just needed to make better choices about what I put inside my body.

I had to rethink the way I thought about food in general. I had to start thinking about food as fuel, because in reality, that is just what food is.

Imagine you have a brand new luxury vehicle. It's shiny and perfect, the most gorgeous shade of cherry red. The wheels are shining, the interior is gleaming, and you just can't wait to take it out for a drive. The thing is, you're out of gas. Now, truly, are you going to go to the pump and pull out the lowest quality gasoline for this wonderful machine? Or would you choose to fill it up with the best quality there is?

When I took this scenario and applied it to my body, I was kind of thrown. Why on earth was I filling my body with low quality food and expecting optimum performance?

This wasn't a "lifestyle" change for me. It was a change of personal mindset.

So how about this? Let's forget all about the word "diet" and just call it Keto from here on out.

Now, let's get down to brass tacks.

I know you're probably thinking, did you say "high fat"? I thought eating fat made you, you know, FAT?

Allow me to explain.

I'm not talking about bad fats, but healthy ones. Yes, there is a difference. There are three major components to how this diet works with the body to make it burn fat for energy instead of relying on the sugar that has been pumped into the tank repeatedly.

First, let me break down how these three components work for the body:

- Protein is processed by the body and broken down into amino acids for proper growth, brain function, hormone regulation, and immunity functions.
- Carbohydrates are broken down into glucose to provide energy for the body. They help maintain blood sugar levels during exercise and help restore muscle glycogen after exercise.
- Fats are made of fatty acids and glycerol and also used to provide energy for the body. Fats are more energy efficient, so the body stores fat to use for later in the case that energy levels run low. There are three main kinds of fat – unsaturated, saturated, and trans. Unsaturated fats are good for you and are usually derived from plants, nuts, seeds, and fish. Saturated fats are better in moderation, and this is the kind of fat you see on red meat and in dairy. Trans fats are to be avoided. These are man-made fats included in processed foods. They increase the risk of disease and affect cholesterol much differently than the other two types.

As you can see, both carbs and fats are used for energy production. So why would I eat more fat if my body stores it for "just in case" scenarios?

The answer lies within the limited carb intake. When the body notices that carbs aren't coming in, it switches to burning fat for fuel.

Our bodies require a lot of energy just to maintain all of its functions, even if we are just sitting still! That means that even if I eat fat with every meal, as long as I limit the carb intake, my body will have to burn my stores of fat just to maintain regular function. That is why I lost weight so effortlessly in the beginning – I had abundant stores of fat!

Comparatively, when I was cutting calories for weight loss, I limited my body's options for energy resources. My body actually entered starvation mode and stubbornly held on to my fat stores in anticipation of going without food.

Our brains are really geared toward survival, so of course it started sending me survival signals. My stomach growled, I craved all kinds of food in large amounts, and I felt lethargic. Cutting calories does work for weight loss eventually, but in the meantime I felt deprived, moody, and very, very hungry. With minimal results, I wasn't motivated to stick with it long-term, and ended up binging on carbs like I was starving.

Picking between these two methods for weight loss was a no brainer for me.

What Do You Mean, No Bread?!

Limiting carb intake means cutting out breads, grains, and starchy vegetables, as well as some high sugar content fruits, sugars, and drinks.

The very first thing I hear when I explain this part is – "I'm not giving up bread! I love bread! I'd rather be able to have my cakes, and doughnuts, and pastries! I'd rather be fat!"

Look, Brenda, I'm not telling you to give up bread for the rest of your dang life.

What I'm trying to explain is that our bodies are really complex, working machines.

I had basically programmed my body to take in bread, break it down for energy, and store the excess in my fat cells in the meantime. In order to break the cycle and reprogram my body, I had to give up bread for a minimum of two weeks at a time, and ideally, do it for four.

Do you think you can do that? Keep a commitment to yourself?

I think you can! So read on!

Carbohydrates are basically turned into sugar for energy, as I went over in the previous chapter. The body breaks them down and stores the excess sugars pulled from the bloodstream as glycogen in the liver. It does all of this to regulate blood sugar levels.

On average, the body stores about 48 hours worth of glycogen in the liver, and then stores the rest of the fat in the body's fat cells. That way, if the liver runs low on glycogen, it can always burn fat for energy.

The main problem is that if carbohydrates are consumed all day, the liver is consistently replenished of its stores, so it never burns the fat. It just stays there and joins all the other fat cells in all their swollen glory.

Are you still with me? Great. Let's keep going.

If the liver uses up all of its stored glycogen and nothing is eaten that can restore it, the body turns to fat stores and starts burning them up for energy. This is why exercise is so commonly linked to weight loss. The body uses up glycogen faster when exercise occurs, then turns to burning fat once it runs out!

However, exercise isn't the only way. As I said, not replenishing the liver's stores also works. Once the body enters ketosis and stays in a fat-burning cycle like this, it literally becomes a walking, talking, fat burning machine by doing nothing more that existing.

Personally, after two weeks of maintaining low glycogen stores in my liver, I was down 15 pounds. I had accomplished what I like to refer to as "The Reset." I had basically confirmed to my wonderful body machine that I would no longer be feeding it carbs for energy, so my body adapted.

Y'all, our bodies are super-adaptable.

Once I had reset my programming, so to speak, my body said, "Oh, okay, I see how it is!" and began burning fat for energy without ever wondering if another doughnut was coming down my pie hole.

You may be wondering, what if another doughnut DOES go down your pie hole?

Simple, guys. I'd simply begin again and reset the programming. The body will go right back to it. Cells have memories. They don't get half as confused as they did the first time around.

Yes, the first time I reset myself, my body was very confused.

I had been a consistent carboholic and eaten carbs at every opportunity, so when my body hit that 48 hour mark, it made me feel a bit funny while it tried to flip the switch over to burning fat for energy. I was dizzy, nauseated, and even a little sweaty while my body tried to adjust.

I happened to have peanut butter cups on hand in my refrigerator. I ate one and felt better within fifteen minutes. Yes, I know that there were carbs consumed there, but not enough to replenish my liver totally. It just helped ease my symptoms in the moment enough for me to say, "I'm good, I'm okay, I'm not dying from lack of sugar."

Once my body had flipped the switch, weight seemed to slide right off of me. I felt clearer, sharper. As it turns out, the brain functions on healthy fats like nobody's business. This is why fish is always referred to as "brain food". It's the Omega-3 fatty acids in fish that help with brain function. That's right! FAT.

Yet the biggest bonus of eating Keto was I NEVER. FELT. HUNGRY.

Seriously, this was like my favorite thing ever. I was hardly ever hungry.

There's a reason for that, too. Protein is more filling, so I felt satisfied for longer periods of time, and the healthy fats I ate were used for energy straight away.

It was the perfect combination for me!

It also eliminated my most hated part of every other diet I had ever tried – being constantly hungry and feeling like a T-Rex that had just been given a side salad to eat while the Velociraptors got to eat whatever they wanted.

Now, my inner T-Rex can eat a steak with melted butter glistening all over the top with a smile on her face and a song in her heart. I could even have a Velociraptor for dessert, guilt-free.

Isn't that awesome?

Electrolyte City

There are side effects to everything, and luckily, I read about this particular one early in my research.

Once the liver starts burning fat for energy, it initiates a reaction from the kidneys. They start flushing out some pretty important electrolytes from the body, like sodium, potassium, and magnesium. Urination increases as the kidneys do their thing, and if the body becomes dehydrated and the electrolytes aren't replaced, it can cause flu-like symptoms.

This is what people refer to as "Keto Flu."

There are hundreds of articles out there dedicated to it. Not everyone experiences it. But before you give up and walk out, hold up just a minute, Greg, and I'll tell you that it doesn't have to be that way.

I'm not big on whining about things. Why complain about something if I can prevent it altogether?

I came up with a game plan ahead of time to prevent myself from experiencing the symptoms – and it worked. Below, I've outlined exactly what I did to avoid Keto Flu symptoms.

1. I drank a lot of water. Carbs bind water to the body, but Keto does the opposite. Water is flushed from the body, so I made sure to stay hydrated!
2. I also drank sugar free electrolyte drinks – these usually have the word "Zero" in the name, to indicate that it's

sugar-free but full of the good stuff.

3. For salt, I consumed some bone-broth, or chicken broth for the sodium. Good grief, this was really easy AND tasty.
4. I started taking supplemental vitamins geared towards replenishing the body of what it was being flushed out – potassium and magnesium.
5. I salted food with sea salt or Himalayan salt. Oh yeah, that's right. I salted it up, buddy. The body NEEDS salt for fluid balance and to prevent dehydration.
6. I ate foods rich in potassium and magnesium. Fish, avocados, and dark chocolate are great sources that also happen to taste great, too.
7. I got some good, solid sleep.

Truly, this is all I needed to do to make Keto Flu a non-issue.

When the body gets what it needs, there is no wasted effort spent on searching the net for answers, getting frustrated, and giving up.

Spare yourself the pain, people! It's not necessary!

Food Lists

Now we come to the greatest question of all – what can I eat on this diet?

I spent weeks looking up different lists compiled by different users online. Some of it was familiar, like almonds and cheddar. Some of it was stuff that had never passed my lips before. What the heck is a chia seed, anyway?!

Finally, I created my own cheat sheet for foods that were familiar to me and that I was comfortable eating. I've outlined this list below, but it is not all inclusive, guys. It's more or less just a starter list. After all, you may know what chia seeds are and love them.

My main goal was to stay under 20 grams of net carbs per day. Sometimes I'd go up to 25, but most of the time, I kept it under 20. This put my body into a state of ketosis and kept my fat flowing right off of me.

Let me explain what I mean by "net" carbs. As it turns out, fiber doesn't count! You know why? Fiber doesn't affect blood sugar levels! If I wanted to eat something with 6g of carbs, and the label said it had 2 g of fiber, then that only counted as 4g carbs toward my daily amount (6-2=4). Quick math!

I read labels, investigated, used that magnificent, beautiful brain of mine and stuck to it. I saw the results on the scale.

Some of the dairy and nuts I have listed have some carb content, but they are low amounts so as long as I kept track and didn't go over my daily allowance, I could still enjoy them.

MEAT

Chicken

Turkey

Duck

Pork

Beef

Shrimp

Crab

Lobster

Clams

Fish

Eggs

DAIRY

Cheese (all kinds)

Cream Cheese

Cottage Cheese

Butter

Sour Cream

Unsweetened Yogurt

Heavy Whipping Cream

FATS

Coconut Oil

Full Fat Mayo

Olive Oil

Butter

Fish Oils

Nut Oils (sunflower, etc.)

Ranch/Blue Cheese Dressing

Eggs

NUTS

Almonds

Walnuts

Pine Nuts

Hazelnuts

Macadamia Nuts

Pecans

VEGETABLES

Asparagus

Celery

Lettuce

Spinach

Cucumber

Zucchini

Cabbage

Cauliflower

Broccoli

Green Beans

Onions

Bell Peppers

FRUITS

Blueberries

Blackberries

Raspberries

Strawberries

Avocados

SNACKS

Pork Rinds

Sunflower Seeds

Olives

Sugar Free Gelatin

Pickles

Pepperoni

Prosciutto

Low Carb Ice Cream

DRINKS

Water

Green Tea

Unsweetened Tea

Almond Milk

Diet Soda

Sugar Free Sports Drinks

Coffee (black)

I got super creative as I went along, and found multiple recipes that worked really well for me. To keep it simple, I included an example of a seven-day meal plan in the back of the book of how I ate and stayed in ketosis, but it's not set in stone. Most people, myself included, prefer a little flexibility. If I woke up and didn't feel like eating eggs, I would just switch it up and eat something else.

I encourage you to get creative with this list. There are about a million more lists out there that cover the same basic criteria; I just wanted to give you a good general overview so you could get an idea of what is regularly consumed on Keto.

Enjoy!

Simple Rules for Grocery Shopping

Believe it or not, I handled this diet by both eating out or staying in and cooking. I'll cover both, but I'm going to start with the grocery store and some simple rules that made shopping a bit easier.

1. I typically stick to the perimeter of the grocery store for the majority of what goes in the cart. Veggies, fruits, dairy, meats – most of all of this is almost always located around the perimeter of the store. This is important to know, because of Rule 2.

2. If it came in a cardboard box, I didn't buy it. If I didn't buy it, I couldn't eat it, and I promise you, you're better off not eating it either. I can feel your resistance from here, but fellas, take a look at those labels. "Food" (and I use that term loosely) that comes in a cardboard box is loaded with preservatives, chemicals, carbohydrates, and sugars to keep it from going bad. You are basically making an argument to eat something that the people selling it KNEW WOULD GO BAD without all that additive crap. Remember what you learned about trans fats? This is where you find the majority of them! Think about that for a minute before moving to the Rule 3 exception.

3. I DID buy canned meats. Tuna, salmon, and even anchovies (if you are so inclined) are awesome Keto staples. Some beef jerky is also cool; I just made sure to review the label. Pepperoni, salami, turkey, roast beef –

guys, I urge you to go to the deli for these to skip the chemicals in the prepackaged type.

4. I bought eggs. And I mean real ones, and a lot of them. Eggs are an incredible food for the body, and the substitute that comes in a carton was just a trip to the bathroom waiting to happen. Unless you've been specifically instructed by a medical professional to avoid them, I say enjoy the real thing.

5. I always buy low-carb tortilla wraps. There are several brands that make them and it makes life easier when I just wanted a dang sandwich or a taco. They are very soft and tasty, too. I honestly can't tell the difference between the low carb and the loaded carb ones. My favorite kind of substitute – the ones that taste like the real thing!

6. Dairy can be a little funny. Low fat options tend to have more carbs than full fat, so substitutions had to be found that fit Keto. I'm a regular coffee drinker and I love cream based soups, so heavy whipping cream became a new source for both. I had to skip over milk and get some almond milk instead. When I bought butter, I had to find REAL butter. No vegetable oil blends, but seriously some full fat, organic, grass-fed butter. This is one switch I didn't mind at all. I had no idea that full fat butter was so dang delicious.

7. CHEESE. Oh my gosh, dear friends, I could eat all kinds of cheese when eating Keto. Cheese does have carbs, but very low amounts, so as long as I was keeping track of it and not digesting an entire block of aged white cheddar (have done it, totally guilty over here), I

could top every meal with cheese totally guilt free – I just had to be careful not to overdo it!

8. Vegetables. Frozen, canned, fresh – are welcome in all forms on Keto, except for two. I had to leave both potatoes and corn behind. Again, like bread, this is not forever. I honestly don't think I could give up sweet potato fries for the rest of my life. BUT I can leave them out of my diet in cycles, and make them the exception, not the norm.

9. Fruit. As it turns out, nature's candy is loaded with natural sugars, meaning that a lot of it is also loaded with carbs. I came up with a simple rule for me to remember what fruits are allowed on Keto: If it ends with the word "berry", it's safe. Strawberries, raspberries, and blueberries – you get the picture.

These rules made it possible for me to quickly shop without issue. I struggled with impulse purchases for a time, because, you know, walking by the bakery with its sweet sugary scent filling the air – it wasn't helping me at all!

I had to modify the way I bought groceries to avoid temptation.

I began making good use of online ordering. Now, I rarely enter the grocery store. I'm a lot more conservative when ordering online, and there are no candy bars calling my name at checkout. It's a win-win!

Mealtime Hacks

This is for all the parents out there, trying to satisfy everyone at the dinner table.

Karen, I see you over there trying to figure out how to tell your carb loving husband that you aren't making mashed potatoes with the meatloaf this time, or explaining to your kids that corn on the cob isn't coming their way any time soon even though it is the only vegetable you can get them to eat with any regularity.

I struggled much the same way at first.

The trick to success in this particular arena was to be ready to modify.

If you're like me, and your kids and spouse have no problem with their weight and you do, they obviously aren't going to give up their PB&J's without a bit of a fuss, and who can blame them?

It was time for a real test of willpower. Could I still have all that carb loaded food on hand for them and say no to it myself? That was the real question.

As it turned out, I had quite a bit of willpower. I just had to have substitutes on hand to make my meal Keto friendly.

The ultimate hack was to be prepared for the eventuality that I would have a slightly different breakfast/lunch/dinner than they did. It wasn't all the time, though. As it turned out, there were some Keto meals that my family loved anyway, so I didn't have to make a substitute every night.

Let me give you some examples of common meals that I substituted certain ingredients for myself to make sure the family was both fed and happy, and I didn't cheat!

1. Spaghetti and Meatballs: Girl, I sure do love some pasta, but it just isn't on the menu for Keto. However, meatballs totally are! I mix 1 pound ground beef with 1-pound Italian sausage and roll into golf ball size balls, baked at 400 degrees for 20 minutes with one rotation halfway through. Spaghetti sauce from a jar can be loaded with extra carbs because of the sugar content, but they make No Sugar Added varieties, so I made sure to have some on hand. While the rest of my family had their carb-loaded noodles, I would buy either spaghetti squash or zoodles (zucchini noodles) frozen from the store. I'd make a plate for myself with zoodles, meatballs, and low carb marinara and top everything with cheese and chow down. No complaints from the peanut gallery on this one.

2. Tacos: Remember those soft shell low carb tortillas I told you I bought? Not a single kid has turned down one in my house. You know why? They can't tell the difference. Taco meat, even fully seasoned, is low carb. I'd top it off with Keto approved taco toppings – cheese, sour cream, tomatoes, onions, peppers, and avocado. I'd leave the beans to the kids and my hubby, but I never felt like I was missing out. Some days, I wasn't feeling the low-carb tortilla vibe, so I'd lay down some romaine lettuce on my plate and top it with taco ingredients – taco salad to the rescue! I'd mix sour

cream and hot sauce to make a kind of dressing – super yummy.

3. Hamburgers: This is one of my favorite things, the all American hamburger. But who wants to look at a little patty on the plate while everyone else has a big, fluffy bun? No, one, that's who. I had to find a way to get a more satisfying bite out of my burger. The answer to this problem was pickles! I'd take my patty and cut it into bite size pieces. Then I'd slice up a whole kosher pickle (my preferred, for the extra crunch). I'd put the pickle on the bottom, put a piece of burger on top, add a slice of cheddar, half of a cherry tomato on top of that, and slide a toothpick down the middle of the stack. Burger kabobs, y'all! I added all kinds of things to change it up, like bacon, lettuce, and avocado. Then I'd dip it into some full fat mayo and mustard and eat my heart out. My kids thought this was so fun, that they now love the burger kabob! This comes in extra handy when I do that thing and completely forget to buy buns for the rest of my family. Oops.

I'm sure you're getting the premise by now. Making substitutions made it possible for me to stay on track without disappointing my family. There are a ton of meals that I didn't even have to modify!

Some days, we'd eat breakfast for dinner: eggs, bacon, sausage, fresh cheese, and some sliced strawberries and I could eat all of it – I just had to lay off the biscuits, waffles, and pancakes.

I'd bake some good old-fashioned chicken, and add a few sides of carb friendly veggies like broccoli and cheese or butternut squash.

I'd grill up some steaks; melt butter all over them, and sauté onions and mushrooms and asparagus to go with it.

There is no rule anywhere that says Keto meals can't be super delicious.

They also do not have to be super complicated.

Don't get me wrong, I love that there are some truly fancy-schmancy bloggers out there that know how to make things taste exactly like the real thing and still be in ketosis, but a lot of those recipes have ingredient lists that are a mile long!

Thanks, but no thanks. I'm a big fan of keeping it simple.

Eating Out

This isn't that much more complicated than modifying meals at home, but I'm going to go through it because we've all been there. A parent-teacher conference that ran late, a football game that went into overtime, the last minute call from our boss that tied us up until 7 – we just don't have time to cook!

So what did I do?

Luckily, Janice, most fast food chains have developed some healthier options so I had choices. This was not half as hard as my brain tried to convince me it was.

I'll start with the easiest substitutes. I'd order whatever the family wanted, but when it came to me, I'd opt for that salad and hold the croutons. I'd get some grilled nuggets and ask for ranch to dip them in. If we were going by a burger joint, I'd ask for extra lettuce and no ketchup on my burger. I'd peel the bun away, wrap everything up in the lettuce and eat it!

You may be wondering, John, about fancier meals; like taking your wife out for sushi. I'd have them hold the rice, order some sashimi and eat my heart out. Seafood is also a great option here, because shrimp, crab, and lobster is all Keto approved, and all I'd have to do is opt for healthier sides or a cream based soup.

I also happen to love any restaurant that has a great steak because, hey, I didn't have to cook it myself!

Again, this all comes down to willpower.

I chose, every day, not to give up.

Some people might say that it was no choice at all, that it was deprivation, but I never felt that way. Every time I stuck to it without giving in, it was like choosing MYSELF. I was choosing ME.

That doesn't mean I didn't have my weak moments. There were definitely some times I'd find myself drooling over what my husband was enjoying on his plate. That was when I'd remind myself that I had cheat days coming.

Yes, you heard me right.

I allowed myself cheat days for every four weeks I stayed in ketosis. I'd take notes of everything I was craving hard. I wanted my cheat days to be full of everything that I was missing the most.

For me, this almost always includes pizza. Man, oh man, do I love pizza.

Some things are worth the wait!

Like seeing downward movement on the scale, and hand-tossed, garlic buttered crust with rich sauce covered with mozzarella, ham, and mushrooms.

I needed those cheat days to provide balance to my life.

I'll tell you how I cheated a little later – for now, let's skip on to how I managed adult beverages without breaking any rules.

Keto Happy Hour

Ah, the moment we've all been waiting for, because sometimes y'all – I need a drink. Either to soothe my frayed nerves or to unwind with some gal pals or to celebrate another wonderful anniversary with my husband, every once in a while, I enjoy a nice trip into the alcoholic beverage section.

On the downside, beer and red wines are both pretty loaded with carbs and sugars.

Does that mean I'm totally out of luck? No, Alice, it sure doesn't.

This is where I had to start getting a little creative to stay in ketosis but still have what I wanted. There are low carb beers and low carb white wines out there, but you really have to pay attention to your serving sizes to make sure you don't top out your maximum carbs for the day.

Pssst. I'm going to tell you a secret.

Unsweetened liquor has hardly any carbs. Uh-huh, yes ma'am, no lie.

I've got to tell you though; drinking straight liquor is pretty nasty. I like a little flavor with my cut-loose, so cocktails are my go-to. Just like with dinners at home and eating out, all I needed were a few modifications to stay on track and still in ketosis. I'm going to list out a few of my favorites here.

First, I'd get prepared by buying what I needed. You know how there are about a zillion flavors on the grocery shelf that you can add to your bottle of water to make it taste yummy with zero calories? Yeah, I'd pick those bad boys up in my favorite flavors for cocktails. Orange is my personal favorite, but strawberry, pineapple, and cranberry are great, too.

Next, I'd buy a big ole bottle of unflavored vodka or rum. I'm sure you can guess why I say unflavored. Wouldn't it be easier with the flavored kind? No, because you can guess how they add that flavor. With sugar! The very thing I'd been working so hard to avoid.

Finally, I'd grab some sugar free gelatin. These make for better daiquiri type drinks than the sugar free flavors for water.

With these ingredients on hand and available, I could whip up a drink anytime I felt like it. Check it out:

1. I'd mix up a bottle of water with orange flavor and shake well. I'd load a large glass with ice and pour a shot of vodka over it, then top it with my orange water. Hello, low-carb screwdriver. If I wanted something a little more rich, I'd add a dash of heavy whipping cream, stir well, and top it with full fat whipped cream. Orange cream cocktail, anyone? Sometimes I'd add one packet of sugar substitute to sweeten it a bit, but this sub takes the edge right off my day, every time!

2. Sometimes I'd want a more summery drink, so pina coladas were the way to go! I'd get pure pineapple extract for this one – the flavor just turns out better. In a blender, I'd mix a cup of ice, a shot glass of rum, a teaspoon of pineapple extract, a packet of sugar

substitute, and a little over 1/3 cup of coconut milk. This one is super yummy.

3. Daiquiris! In a blender, I'd add ice, rum, and any flavor of sugar free gelatin. Sometimes I'd play with the amounts of liquor, depending on how buzzed I wanted to be. Once I'd nailed my combo, I'd pour it into a glass and top it with full fat whipped cream.

4. Let's not leave the classics out. Unsweetened rum and diet soda still works, and takes about five seconds to make.

I was happy to discover that there was little I had to do to stay in ketosis and still have a little fun.

Cheater, Cheater

For the love of all that's holy, I made it.

I successfully stuck to Keto for four weeks. I weigh less and feel great.

Yet, I really, really, really want to eat a dang muffin. And some pizza. And possibly some birthday cake, doughnuts, and a roll, and maybe a biscuit, too.

So let's talk about why I would cheat after all that hard work, Richard, because if we don't, you may think I simply jumped the track entirely and put back on all the weight I'd lost plus some!

I allow myself cheat days because if I don't, I'm much more likely to slide back into old habits that don't serve me. If I don't indulge every once in a while, it's easy to justify one little thing here and there, until I've upped my carb intake for almost every single day. Putting my cheat days right out front, where everyone can see them, gives me the freedom to say when and how I'll cheat, and puts a deadline on how long. Then I jump right back into Keto with no issue, because I know I'll have another cheat soon enough.

After all, I'm still losing weight. It took a long time for me to put all those pounds on, so I put no pressure on myself to lose it all in one month. It just isn't going to happen. It's a lot easier to set a little mini goal, like ten pounds, and work my four weeks and then take a little break and have my cheat days, then set my next goal and continue on. This totally makes the entire process more manageable.

I do like to give myself a time frame, as I mentioned earlier, so I usually cheat for four days, followed by a three day fast to get back into ketosis. Then I begin my next four-week Keto journey. That's one week in between each stretch that I look forward to every single time.

So, it's day one of cheat day. How do I spend it?

Thoughts of bread, biscuits, gravy, french fries, or even a big old fashioned baked potato loaded with all the options usually fill my head. I plan it all out, and I am almost always amazed at what happens.

I quickly discover that I can't consume as much as I used to be able to nosh on. That is because in those four weeks, I've trained my stomach to handle smaller portions because protein and fat just don't take up that much room in the stomach. It's a fun little side effect.

A not-so-fun side effect is that my bowel doesn't handle these carb-laden foods as easily either. Again, remember that I reprogrammed my body for better fuel. Now, I'm clogging up the gas tank with a hefty dose of sugar.

Boy howdy, cheating is not quite as easy as I thought it was going to be.

I had to moderate myself and not go completely crazy, because my body simply couldn't handle it!

I used to be able to eat an entire medium pizza all by myself, in my carboholic days. Now, on my cheat days, I can only manage that if I order thin crust, and I still feel overstuffed afterwards. I feel better if I stick to half.

What I'm getting at here is that when I cheat, I don't sit down with a box of 50 donut holes and go to town. I eat the same breakfast I normally would, but I let myself have a biscuit. I have a thick reuben sandwich for lunch on marbled rye bread. When I eat dinner, I may eat some fried chicken with mashed potatoes. I don't over-do it; I just eat until I'm full.

It works out better this way, because my body handles it a bit better, and I get to enjoy some things I've missed eating.

I also steadfastly remind myself during this time that four days off of Keto will not undo four weeks of steady work towards weight loss. The most I've ever gained was three pounds during my cheat period. It came right back off right after I completed a fast, which basically means that it's water weight anyway!

Speaking of fasts, read on, my brothers and sisters of weight loss! I cover that next.

Fasts

When most people hear the word "fast" in relation to dieting, they think in terms of no food whatsoever and that gnawing, hungry yuck that comes with it.

That is NOT what I'm talking about, Sally. A keto fast is simply a removal of my carb allowance of 20 g a day, and drinking a load of water to rid my body of all evidence of my cheating. It can be done!

There are a couple of ways to do this, and I'm going to go over all three. I've done them all, and they all work.

1. The Egg Fast – Basically, this is exactly what it sounds like. I eat eggs for three days. Now there is a lot of data out there for this particular fast, as in how often to eat an egg (once every 3 hours) and to always pair it with an equal amount of fat. If one egg seemed like too little to hold me over, I'd eat two.

I also switched the menu up a little, because as we all know there are tons of ways to enjoy eggs. Here are some of my faves:

- Fried egg in 1 tbsp. of butter
- Boiled egg with one teaspoon mayo
- Two devilled egg halves
- Scrambled egg with one ounce of cheese

I drank water all day, and before I knew it, I was a fat burning machine once more!

1. Meat & Fat Fast – I recommend using ground meat for this, but only because it is easily measured. You can have 1 cup of ground meat at a time, paired with healthy fat for three days. Some examples are below:

- 1 cup ground beef with 3 teaspoons of butter melted on top
- 1 cup taco meat with 3 teaspoons of butter melted on top
- 1 cup ground turkey with one ounce of cheddar sprinkled on top.
- 1 cup sausage with one ounce of cheddar on top

Again, I flushed my system with water.

1. The Combination Fast – I'll be truthful with you. I made this one up myself. It follows the same guidelines as the first two, except you can switch up the meals. Eat an egg with a healthy fat in the morning, a cup of beef with fat at lunchtime, and have 1 cup of tuna, with mayo, and topped with boiled egg for dinner. You can move it around whichever way you like, but the results are nearly the same. This helps keep me from going crazy by eating only one kind of meal for three days. This one is the one I do most often, and I find it works just as well, if not better, than the first two. Hey, did I mention drinking water? Seriously – hydration is the

most important thing during a fast. I drank and drank water like crazy.

Just like before, these fasts helped me to accomplish a quick Reset by getting rid of the stores of glycogen in my liver that built up with my cheat days. I did make sure to have a peanut butter cup on hand and ready just in case I experienced another Crash. I very rarely end up using it though.

Personally, the first time it happened to me was the worst. My body is now so adapted to Keto that it doesn't even panic at low glycogen stores. It already knows what to do.

Intermittent Fasting

I feel like this is a good time to cover Intermittent Fasting, because at one point or another in any diet, I would run into the dreaded weight loss stall, or plateau.

Don't panic, Paul! There are a couple of different reasons for stalls in weight loss, and I'm going to tell you what I did to break through them.

First, let me tell you about hidden sugars and dairy.

Up to this point, I had clung on to my diet sodas and used all of my carb allowance for cheese just because I love it so much.

Yet the fact remains that diet soda still has artificial sweeteners in it, and cheese can be pretty loaded with carbs it's being eaten all the time.

Sure enough, when I gave up the soda and cut way back on the cheese, my weight loss picked back up. Bummer.

I see the look you are all giving me. You said you got to eat cheese!

I did. I still do! Yet I had to admit that sometimes I took it to far, and the result was a plateau. That's not what I wanted.

I can still offer you hope, sweet friends. There is another option to cutting out diet sodas and cheese completely: Intermittent Fasting. I started doing a 16/8 fasting schedule, meaning that I consumed all of my calories from food within 8 hours, and fasted for the other 16.

This may not sound like very much fun, but for about 8 hours of that fast, I was sleeping and wasn't eating anyway, so it wasn't that hard to pull this schedule off. I will also tell you this – every time I stalled on my weight loss journey, Intermittent Fasting broke the stall.

So how did I do it?

I wake up at 5:30 am almost every day. For the first six hours of my day, I drink coffee or water. At 11:30 am, I start my eight-hour stretch of calorie intake. I eat a wonderful keto lunch around that time, have a few snacks, and make sure I eat my dinner before 7:30. Then I have either some herbal tea or water after that, but no more food. I go to bed by 10 pm, and continued this cycle until I broke through my plateau.

The reason it works is because A.) I was consuming fewer calories and I was already in a fat burning metabolic state and B.) Insulin levels drop when no food is eaten, so my body would ramp up the burning of my stored fat for energy.

You may be surprised to learn there are people that do fasts on a much stricter schedule. This is just what worked for me, so I stuck with it whenever I hit a roadblock to my weight loss.

Recap

I feel like it's necessary to sum it all up here. Once you've read this little guidebook through, you may just like a handy-dandy little page to flip to that summarizes the main points.

- Eating Keto essentially means eating really healthy whole foods that aren't packaged and are super low in carbohydrates. Food = fuel for the body. Take care of your body, because you only get one!
- It's NOT forever. However, I discovered that I might want it to be. I never noticed how heavily bread sat in my stomach until I stopped eating it. Now, when I cheat, I can feel how heavy and bloated it makes me feel.
- There are side effects if the body becomes dehydrated and electrolytes are not replenished. Drinking water is really, really important.
- Health is not something you can buy. Everything comes down to choices. I simply started making choices to help my body become more efficient at burning my fat stores.
- Avoiding processed, packaged "food" will have benefits. Again, ewww. Just don't. It's not worth it. Our bodies are worthy of better food, better fuel. Don't forget that.
- Modifying meals to stay on track is the way to go. There is nothing that can't be managed without good planning and a good attitude. Even pulling through a

drive-thru, I know I've got this.

- Drink and be merry. I simply avoid beer, which by the way, comes from grains. Liquor is easier. Oh, and I don't drink and drive. Not because Keto has anything to do with that, but because it's a bad idea in general.
- Cheating from time to time is okay. I never let myself feel deprived. One time I was craving pecan pie so bad I was dreaming about eating it! I went and had a slice and then jumped right back on the wagon. It's okay! It wasn't the end of the world.
- Fast to Reset the liver into fat burning mode. It's quick and easy. I can do this so easily now, I don't even think about it. It's only 3 days! That is not very long!
- Weight loss plateaus can be broken by using Intermittent Fasting or by cutting back on diet sodas and dairy.

One other thing I did before I started was measuring my arms, calves, waist, hips, and thighs in inches. This was a fantastic way to see success when the pounds on the scale weren't moving fast enough for me. It's amazeballs.

Finally, I want to remind you that I did all of this for myself, no one else. I wanted to feel better in my skin, wear regular sized clothes, reduce my health risks, and feel good about me. I was the poster child for failed diets. I know how hopeless it can feel, and I can honestly say I no longer feel that way at all.

If you walk away from this book with anything, I really, truly want it to be hope. My success also means that you, too, can have success should you choose to consult your doctor and give it a shot.

With much love to my fellow carboholics,

Christina D. Ford

Seven-Day Meal Plan

Below you will find a seven-day meal plan that has a lot of different options that I regularly use when trying to switch it up so I don't get bored with the same meals over and over.

To be completely honest, I rarely have a week that is this varied. I just wanted to show you all the different ways that it can be done, whereas in reality, it isn't so unusual for me to eat boiled eggs every single day for breakfast because I'm tired and I simply don't want to give it more thought!

There are also times that I get sick of eggs in the mornings and switch to microwave bacon out of convenience. I do a lot in the way of making things as simple as I can for myself, because the harder it is for me to prepare it, the less likely I am to stick to it.

The majority of the lunches I have listed here are simple enough to pack up in advance, and I do that to make it easy for me to grab and go in the mornings. I usually spend some time on Sunday prepping lunches for the week so I never have to think about it when I'm busy trying to get my kids out of the door on a school day.

You will notice that I have a lot of drinks listed, and that is so I remember to stay hydrated. I drink a lot of hot green tea, for instance, because it has many health benefits and has been linked with weight loss numerous times. I also drink a lot of water. My coffee recipes vary depending on what I'm in the mood for, and you will see I have several options that I use to add flavor.

The dinners I have listed are easily made and are regular alternates in my meal planning. I tried to list some of the tastiest options I use, because it makes me look forward to dinner and eating something delicious. I enjoy every single dinner I have laid out here on a regular basis.

Finally, I included some easy and simple desserts. Again, there are recipes out there for those that want to go the extra mile to have something sweet ready and waiting, but I find I do better when I can just have a little low carb friendly ice cream or yogurt now and then. I don't eat dessert every day. Sometimes I crave it, sometimes I don't. I just have the options ready for when I do, so I don't catch myself with my fingers in the kid's cookie jar.

Day 1:

Breakfast: 2 eggs scrambled in butter with a sprinkle of cheddar cheese on top, coffee with 1 tbsp. heavy whipping cream and a dash of sugar free vanilla syrup.

Mid-morning drink: Hot green tea with one packet of sugar substitute

Lunch: Grilled Chicken Caesar Salad – no croutons – with Caesar dressing, with water to drink

Snack: Almonds, more water

Dinner: New York Strip pan-fried in butter, asparagus, diet green tea

Dessert: ½ cup low carb ice cream

Day 2:

Breakfast: 2 boiled eggs, salted and peppered, with one oz. white cheddar. Blended iced coffee – 1 cup ice, 1 cup coffee, and 1 cup unsweetened vanilla coconut milk. Add sugar free syrup for extra flavor if needed.

Mid-morning drink: Diet Green Tea

Lunch: Tuna with mayo, mustard, salt, pepper, and diced jalapenos in a low carb tortilla, water

Snack: Spicy pork rinds and sugar free sports drink

Dinner: Grilled chicken breast with broccoli and cheese, water

Dessert: 5 strawberries sliced, topped with full fat whipped cream

Day 3:

Breakfast: 2 sausage patties smeared with guacamole, coffee with sugar free creamer

Mid-morning drink: Hot green tea with one packet of sugar substitute

Lunch: BLT salad – no croutons - with ranch dressing and sliced avocado, 1 bottle of electrolyte water

Snack: A cheese stick and pepperoni slices, diet green tea

Dinner: Taco in low carb tortilla wrap, seasoned ground beef, tomatoes, sour cream, shredded cheddar, water to drink

Dessert: sugar free gelatin with full fat whipped cream

Day 4:

Breakfast: Microwaved bacon and a devilled egg, coffee with unsweetened almond milk and a dash of sugar free caramel syrup

Mid-morning drink: Sugar free sports drink

Lunch: Leftover taco meat on a bed of romaine, topped with shredded cheddar, tomatoes, avocado, and sour cream and hot sauce, water

Snack: Prosciutto, diet green tea

Dinner: Mock alfredo with sautéed shrimp and asparagus (using zoodles instead of noodles and 1 cup heavy whipping cream mixed with 1/3 cup grated parmesan cheese and pressed garlic to make sauce), water

Dessert: Handful of raspberries/blackberries

Day 5:

Breakfast: 2 egg omelet with shredded cheddar cheese and spinach, iced coffee with 1 cup ice, 1 cup coffee, 1 cup unsweetened coconut milk

Mid-morning drink: Hot green tea with 1 packet of sugar substitute

Lunch: Ham, turkey, and cheese roll-ups, 1 bottle of electrolyte water

Snack: Whole kosher dill pickle, diet green tea

Dinner: Buffalo chicken dip (the kind made with cream cheese and shredded chicken), with cucumber slices to dip like chips or celery sticks, water

Dessert: Low-carb full fat yogurt

Day 6:

Breakfast: 1 fried egg with sausage patty and 1 ounce slice of cheddar, coffee with sugar free creamer

Mid-morning drink: Sugar free sports drink

Lunch: Chicken salad with celery, red onion, and full fat mayo in a low carb tortilla wrap, diet green tea

Snack: Olives with crumbled feta, water

Dinner: Grilled salmon with BLT side salad with ranch dressing, water

Dessert: ½ cup low carb vanilla ice cream with a few blueberries on top

Day 7:

Breakfast: 1 fried egg in 1 tbsp. butter, a slice of Canadian bacon, coffee with 1 tbsp. heavy whipping cream and a dash of sugar free vanilla syrup.

Mid-morning drink: Hot green tea with 1 packet of sugar substitute

Lunch: Grilled chicken nuggets dipped in ranch dressing, diet green tea

Snack: 2 devilled egg halves, water

Dinner: Philly cheese steak (shredded beef, sautéed bell peppers, mozzarella) stuffed mushrooms, electrolyte water

Dessert: Low carb full fat yogurt